YOUR BODY

YOUR MIND

&

YOUR DIET

*Lose That Weight, Get Rid of Diabetes And
Settle For A Happy Life*

John J. Saldini

TABLE OF CONTENT

CHAPTER SIX

ELIMINATION DIET
DIETARY FOODS TO AVOID   2
WHAT CAN YOU CAN EAT

INTRODUCTION

It's no secret that eating healthy feels good. But why is this the case? How does the food we eat have such a significant impact on how we function day today?

When it comes to our health, the foods we put into our bodies can have a big impact, especially on our hearts. Obesity, weight gain, inactivity, stress, high blood pressure, high cholesterol, and obesity are all associated with an increased risk of heart disease and cancer.

When you get home from a long day at work, it's tempting to order food or order takeout and unwind. When you're fatigued, who wants to go through the hassle of cooking and cleaning? While occasionally eating fast food isn't harmful, doing so on a regular basis might lead to an unhealthy diet. Unhealthy eating habits might be harmful to your health in the long run.

When we ingest something, it passes through a digestive process. This includes absorbing vitamins and minerals from food and transferring them through the bloodstream to the blood vessels, coronary arteries, and heart muscle.

Your heart might pump harder and exert more energy depending on the foods you eat. This could lead to heart failure and a heart attack in the future.

The amount of salt you consume has a significant impact on your heart rate and blood pressure. When you eat salty foods, your body retains water to dilute the volume of blood This causes your heart to work harder as more blood circulates throughout your body.

A daily salt consumption of 180 to 500 mg is considered safe. However, the average American consumes more than 3,400 mg of sodium each day. The majority of these are processed and pre-prepared foods.

Saturated and trans fats elevate poor cholesterol and can lead to arterial hardening and plaque formation on the inner linings of blood vessels, restricting them even further. Because the apertures are restricted, the heart has to work harder to maintain blood flow and pump blood through the narrowed channels.

Likewise, not eating a nutritious diet may increase your risk of cancer. While some of these foods may be hazardous to your health and heart function, others may be beneficial. Olive oil and whole grains, for example, can help decrease cholesterol and prevent plaque formation in the arteries. Your heart will be able to pump blood more efficiently, resulting in less strain and blood that lacks the nutrients we require. These foods are high in fat, sugar, and salt while lacking in fiber and vitamins. If you are concerned about your calorie intake, consult your doctor or nutrition and dietetics professional.

CHAPTER ONE

What is Poor Nutrition?

Depriving our bodies of the nutrients they require can result in poor nutrition and eating habits, which can lead to obesity, diabetes, and increased risk factors for stroke, heart disease, and cancer.

Putting the wrong kinds of food in your body leads to poor nutrition. These foods are high in fat, sugar, and salt while being lacking in fiber and vitamins

Overeating can also contribute to poor nutrition. Even if you eat the right foods, ingesting more calories per day than you burn can lead to weight gain and obesity. Diabetes and heart disease are linked to obesity and being overweight or obese. Anorexia and bulimia patients, for example, are just as vulnerable to heart disease and other illnesses as those who overeat.

The body's effect of insufficient nutrition

Poor nutrition can have a variety of effects on your health, including mental health, energy levels, complexion, and overall well-being. In the short term, a poor diet might increase tension, fatigue, and our ability to concentrate.

• dental decay

• high blood pressure

• high cholesterol

• heart disease and stroke

• type 2 diabetes

• osteoporosis

• some malignancies

• depression

• eating disorders

Poor nutrition can have a negative impact on your daily health and well-being, as well as your ability to enjoy and participate in activities.

We've all heard that eating healthy may alter your life and make you live longer and more active. But what really is healthy eating, and how can you start putting it into practice and changing unhealthy habits? Some people want to lose weight, while others want to lower blood pressure, and still, others just want to live a healthy lifestyle. This change will not take place. This is hardly an overnight transformation. You can't just break all of your bad habits on Sunday morning and not have cravings. This is a steady process that might begin with a simple substitution of steamed broccoli for loaded mashed potatoes as a side dish. For a mid-morning snack, go for an apple rather than chips.

Here are some helpful hints and suggestions that will have you on your way to bursting with health and vigor in no time:

• Increase your daily fruit and vegetable consumption. A bowl of blueberry oatmeal is a delicious way to start the day. Aim for two servings of fruit per day and five servings of veggies per day.

 But what really is healthy eating, and how can you begin implementing it and breaking unhealthy habits?

• Reduce your sodium intake.

Make a conscious effort to use less and less salt on your food until you just need a dash.

• Reduce your sugar intake.

Avoid sugary snacks by replacing sugar with honey in your coffee.

If you're looking for something sweet, consider combining frozen bananas and strawberries.

• Increase your water intake by half your body weight in ounces.

Water, rather than sugary drinks, can help you lose weight, and clear your complexion, and because our bodies are 70% water, you may feel healthier overall.

• Keep track of your portions.

Half of your dinner plate should be filled with a variety of vegetables or salad, and the other half should be filled with lean protein meals like meat, fish, poultry, or legumes (chickpeas, for example).

Prepare in advance.

People eat fast food or a bag of chips for a variety of reasons, one of which is that they are in a hurry.

On weekends, plan your meals, including snacks, and buy only what you need and prepare your food.

Not only will this help you eat healthier, but it will also help you save money.

If you're worried about your eating habits, talk to your doctor or a dietician nutritionist about your alternatives.

The foods we put into our bodies enable our cells to carry out their essential jobs. Consider it like growing a garden. For the greatest results, utilize the proper soil and the right quantity of sunlight when sowing tomato seeds. If you use cheap dirt and don't expose it to adequate sunlight, it will die. you'll get a tomato, but it won't be the ripest, roundest, reddest, or tastiest tomato.

To put it another way, providing our bodies with the proper nutrients can assist us in becoming a healthier version of ourselves. This way of thinking about food It goes beyond calories and the distinction between good and bad meals. You should focus on the foods you eat rather than the foods you avoid.

Consider eating as a means of nourishing your body and preventing cardiovascular disease.

A faulty diet can cause malnutrition, poor digestion, inflammation, undesirable weight gain, and obesity. It can also harm your mental health and increase your risk of developing chronic conditions like diabetes and heart disease.

12

CHAPTER TWO

What Constitutes a Healthy Diet?

As you've probably heard a million times, eat a well-balanced diet. But what is a well-balanced diet, exactly? These simple items make up a well-balanced diet and can help you avoid a range of health concerns if you stick to the recommended serving sizes.

An unhealthy diet can include excessive use of specific food or substance.

A high-sodium diet is an example of this.

If you eat bacon, cold cuts, and other salt-preserved foods on a daily basis, you're probably receiving too much sodium.

This can lead to a range of health problems, including high blood pressure and an increased risk of cardiovascular disease.

While a pinch of salt here and there may not seem like a huge concern, 9 out of 10 Americans consume too much salt.

In general, eating too much of anything can lead to a poor diet with bad health consequences.

Unhealthy Eating Pose Risks

Unhealthy eating habits can result in obvious changes such as acne, bloating, and weight gain. Certain bad diets, such as those associated with too much fast food, can lead to obesity and related diseases. Obesity increases the risk of diabetes, heart disease, osteoarthritis, stroke, and a variety of other illnesses, although not everyone's weight causes physical changes. However, just because the repercussions of bad eating habits are not immediately obvious does not mean they do not occur.

It's possible to eat an unhealthy diet for a long time and then feel the consequences. Malnutrition is primarily caused by junk food and fast food. Malnutrition is one of the most serious consequences of poor eating habits, and it can lead to diseases like scurvy. Scurvy is a vitamin C deficit that can affect persons who eat a carbohydrate-rich diet and shun fresh fruits and vegetables. A bad diet does not induce scurvy. You'd have to be vitamin C deficient for three months to get this illness.

Long-term repercussions of nutrient shortages are possible. Certain vitamins and minerals can lessen the risk of disorders that arise later in life, such as osteoporosis, Nutritional Sciences. Calcium and vitamin D are important for bone health and can help you avoid osteoporosis as you become older.

Your dietary choices have far more consequences than you may know. Because your digestive system contains billions of microorganisms, every meal you eat has the potential to modify your gut microbiota, just like your digestive system contains trillions of microbes. The bacteria that live in these communities are influenced by the foods you eat on a daily basis. Poor diets can disturb microbial communities., allowing too many of one species to invade your gastrointestinal system. This can cause problems with digestion and metabolism, as well as diseases like inflammatory bowel disease. Your food can affect your mental health since a cranial nerve connects your gut to your brain.

Eating habits might have a bigger impact than you think. Understanding the short- and long-term consequences of poor eating habits is critical, as is striving for a well-balanced diet.

Diabetes and Weight Loss
Diabetes is a challenging disease to manage, and a poor diet just makes matters worse. A nutritious diet is required to keep blood glucose levels in the proper range, which is critical for diabetics. how

In brief

People with diabetes are overweight or obese in almost 90% of cases. Weight loss slows the progression of diabetic problems, whereas obesity and excess weight exacerbate insulin resistance. Doctors must know how to treat diabetic patients with obesity, Because of the increased risk of diabetic complications in obese individuals, treatment may include counseling and behavioral management, as well as referral to a weight-loss program and medication delivery.

However, if you have diabetes, there are some benefits to lowering weight if you are overweight.

You'll have more energy and your risk of significant problems such as heart disease and stroke will be reduced. Losing weight might also aid with diabetes management. Furthermore, if you have type 2 diabetes, decreasing weight may result in diabetic remission.

Millions of people with diabetes, on the other hand, struggle to maintain a healthy weight. You are not alone, and assistance is available; a wise first step is to seek assistance and guidance from your healthcare team.

Overweight or obese patients account for 60% of type 1 diabetes patients and 85% of type 2 diabetes patients.

The Advantages of Decreasing Weight
Losing weight has a variety of physical and psychological benefits.

If you acquire weight around your waist, fat can accumulate around your organs, such as your liver and pancreas. This could cause an issue called insulin resistance.

As a result, decreasing weight may aid the proper functioning of the insulin you manufacture or inject have significant health advantages If you have obesity, losing 15kg (or 2 stone 5lbs) as fast and securely as possible after your diagnosis will increase your chances of putting your diabetes into remission. This could mean fully stopping your diabetes medication, which could be life-changing. If you lose weight quickly and close to your diagnosis, this is far more likely. It's a fallacy that losing weight slowly is healthier.

The majority of people say they are happier, have more energy, and sleep better.

There is also a lot of information to help you remain on track and avoid gaining weight by helping you maintain a healthy weight.

If you have diabetes and use insulin or a sulphonylurea, your doctor may need to evaluate your prescription as you lose weight and become more active.

It may be essential to reduce the dose or make other adjustments but first, visit your doctor.

Some people wish to lose weight so that they don't have to take as many diabetes drugs. If you have type 2 diabetes, losing 5% of your body weight can help decrease your blood pressure and cholesterol.

This can have a big impact on your overall health and help you prevent serious illnesses like heart disease and stroke.

CHAPTER THREE

Why Strive for weight Loss?

Before you begin, you must first determine what constitutes a healthy weight and the numbers you wish to achieve and figure out your BMI and waist circumference.

Understanding Your Weight.

Accordingly, the more weight you shed, the better your health will be, but even decreasing 5% of your excess weight will help.

BMI calculates your weight and height to see if you're at a healthy weight it does not consider how much fat you have around your middle, you must also measure your waist. You can use the NHS calculator to calculate your BMI, which will show you your ideal weight range.

Obesity makes it difficult for many people to have a healthy BMI.

Determine your waist circumference.

Gender and ethnicity both influence your waist size.

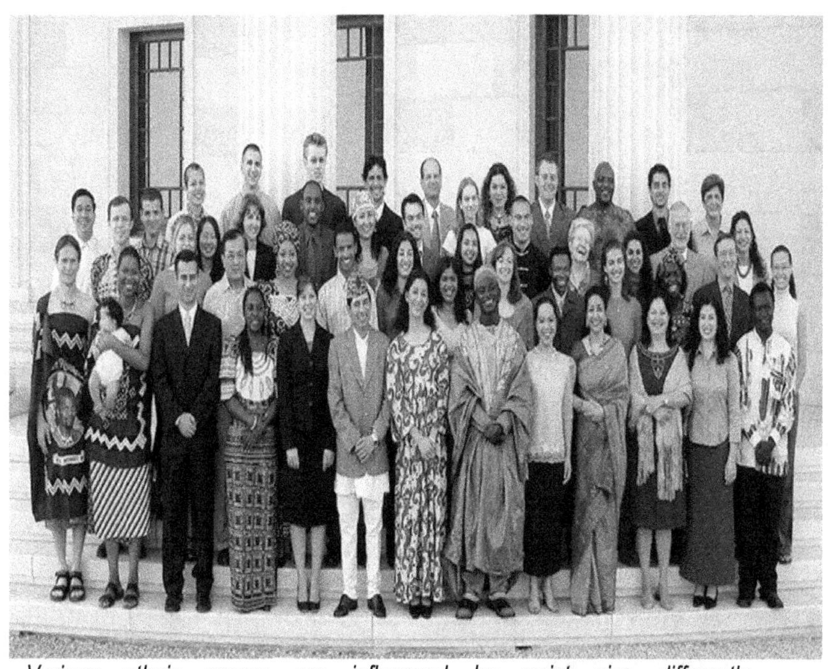

Various ethnic groups are influenced by waist size differently

• It should be less than 80cm for all ladies (31.5in)

• The majority of men are under 94cm (37in) tall.

• Guys from South Asia must be under 90cm tall (35in).

Can Diabetes Make You Gain Weight?

If you have type 1 diabetes and begin using insulin, you may gain weight. This can be due to a variety of factors, including the amount of insulin you take, your food, and the type of insulin you're using.

Insulin is a growth hormone, and taking any growth hormone will cause you to gain weight. When you're diagnosed with diabetes, one of the signs is rapid weight loss, and weight gain is a normal part of the healing process.

The type of insulin you use might have a variety of effects on your weight. We have more information on the various sorts and how they can affect you.

Weight loss diets for diabetics

You may have heard that diabetes can be managed with dietary changes. There are many ways to reduce weight, but there is no such thing as a one-size-fits-all diet. It all begins with determining how to take fewer calories than you need.

A calorie (or kcal) is a measure of energy found in food and beverages.

Everything you do in your body uses energy, from breathing to sleeping to exercising.

When you eat, you replace the energy you've absorbed, which helps you maintain a healthy weight.

According to government estimates, men require around 2,500kcal per day to maintain a healthy weight, while women require around 2,000kcal per day. Most people, however, require different calorie amounts based on how their bodies work, how active they are, and any weight management goals they have.

There are 7-day meal plans available to help you lose weight. They're all Approved, nutritionally balanced, and calorie and carbohydrate count, and they can help you lose weight:

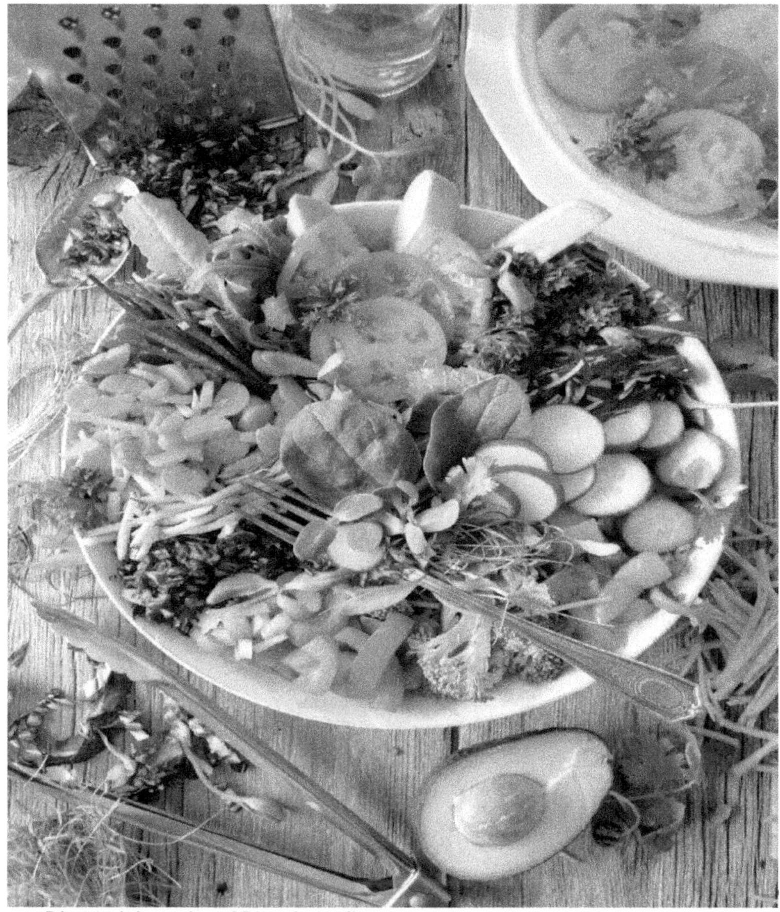

Direct trial used an 850-calorie diet

• *Low-carb diet plan Mediterranean plan*

• Diet regimens with fewer calories, such as 1,200 or 1,500 calories each day

The best method is the one you're most likely to stick to, according to research. The idea is to find a plan that you like and that works for

Diets with Very Low Calories

A low-calorie diet contains between 800 and 1200 calories per day; the Direct trial used an 850-calorie diet.

An extremely low-calorie diet is defined as eating less than 800 calories per day. The construct of low- or very-low-calorie meal plans was not intended here because most people would find these difficult to prepare at home. The majority of people who follow these diets consume nutritionally adequate meal replacement products such as soups and smoothies. If you want to attempt a low-calorie diet like the one in Direct, talk to your doctor or nurse first, especially if you take insulin or other medications.

Other eating plans

Although a low Glycemic index (GI) diet can help you manage your blood sugar levels, but there is little evidence that it can assist people with diabetes to lose weight.

The Paleo diet and intermittent fasting (such as the 5:2 diet) are two other popular diets.

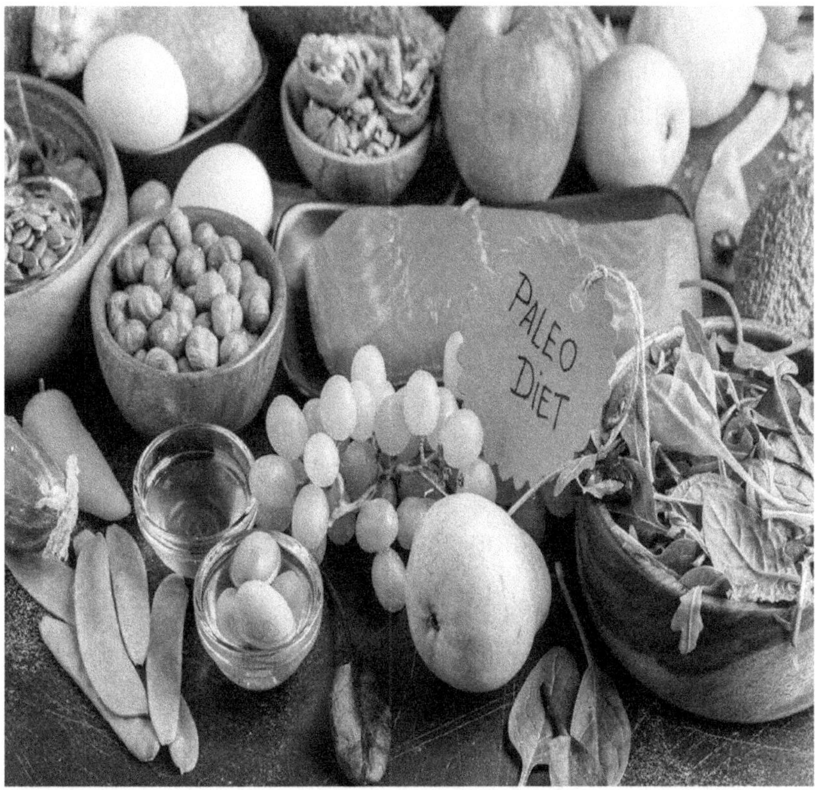

a paleo diet and intermittent fasting are good eating plans to help lose some of that weight

Unfortunately, there is little evidence to claim that these are useful for weight loss in diabetics.

Weight-Loss Regimens Sold Commercially

Some people decide to join a commercial weight-loss program because they feel they need extra support.

Calorie-controlled diets or meal replacements, such as milkshakes or bars, are common.

It's critical to ask a lot of questions about these programs so that you have all of the data and information you need to make an educated decision.

Here are some suggestions:

•Was a healthcare practitioner involved in any way?

• Does the program provide diabetes advice (particularly if you're at risk of hypos)?

• Is this program providing you with all of the nutrients you require?

• Is the program supportive and educational?

If you want, you can try one of these meal plans or another type of diet, you must first explore your options with your diabetes team.

Because changing your diet will have an impact on your medicine or blood sugar levels, you'll need their guidance and assistance.

CHAPTER FOUR

Top Weight Loss Habits to Break

Did you know that forming a habit takes 21 days?

Also, did you know that it takes 21 days to break a bad habit?

It's crucial to remember that minor changes can make a significant effect, particularly if you're trying to reduce weight.

A few minor tweaks to your everyday eating choices and routines can often make a big difference.

1. Meal Skipping

Breakfast, lunch, and supper are the best times to eat since they keep your energy levels and hunger hormones in check.

If you skip meals, you'll eat more later in the day.

You will crave high-calorie, high-fat, low-nutrition items if you go more than 3-4 hours without eating.

2. Eating Out

It can be challenging to put yourself in certain situations when you are first trying to reduce weight.

Instead of eating out, prepare your meals ahead of time.

People who dine out regularly are more likely to be overweight, consume more fat and sugar, and engage in less physical activity, according to studies. It doesn't matter if it's fast food or a five-star establishment.

When we go out to eat, we eat more food and take in more calories. However, if you do have to eat, out check out this

We all know that eating out may be a time bomb when it comes to keeping to a balanced diet.

According to surveys, the food you eat when you're not at home is nutritionally inferior to the meals you prepare and consume at home in every aspect.

Sticking to a healthy eating plan, on the other hand, does not necessitate avoiding eating out.

Eating Ideas to Keep You on Track:

1. Make your own decisions.

When requesting menu adjustments, be aggressive. For example, if an item is fried, ask for it to be grilled instead. if a meal comes with a side of chips, request that it be replaced with vegetables or salad.

These queries are asked more frequently than you might imagine, and the restaurant will usually comply without reluctance.

2. Do things your way.

When requesting menu adjustments, be aggressive. For example, if an item is fried, ask for it to be grilled instead, if a meal comes with a side of chips, request vegetables or salad instead.

These queries are requested more frequently than you might imagine, and the restaurant will usually comply without reluctance.

3. Double the number of vegetables.

A side of veggies in a restaurant is frequently more of a modest garnish—a carrot and a slice of cucumber, for example.

Request two or three times the usual amount of vegetables when ordering and offer to pay more.

(Occasionally, they will not even charge you!)

4. Cut in half.

Before your main dish arrives at the table, request that it be halved and packed, or share a main course with your dining companion.

Restaurants frequently provide two to three times the standard serving size.

5. Select two appetizers.

If the appetizer menu at a restaurant appeals to you, order two as a main course rather than an entree.

Choose an appetizer of seafood or grilled meat, as well as a veggie.

That is frequently enough food to satisfy you.

6. Dip the fork in the sauce.

The greatest recommendation is to serve the dressing with a salad.

On the side, ask for a tiny bowl of dressing. Using an empty fork, dip a salad forkful into the dressing and skewer it. You'll be surprised at how similar this tastes and how little dressing you'll need, resulting in a significant reduction in calories.

7. Think forward. Before you go, look over the menu. This is something we always tell our clients to do! Most restaurants' menus are available on their websites; have

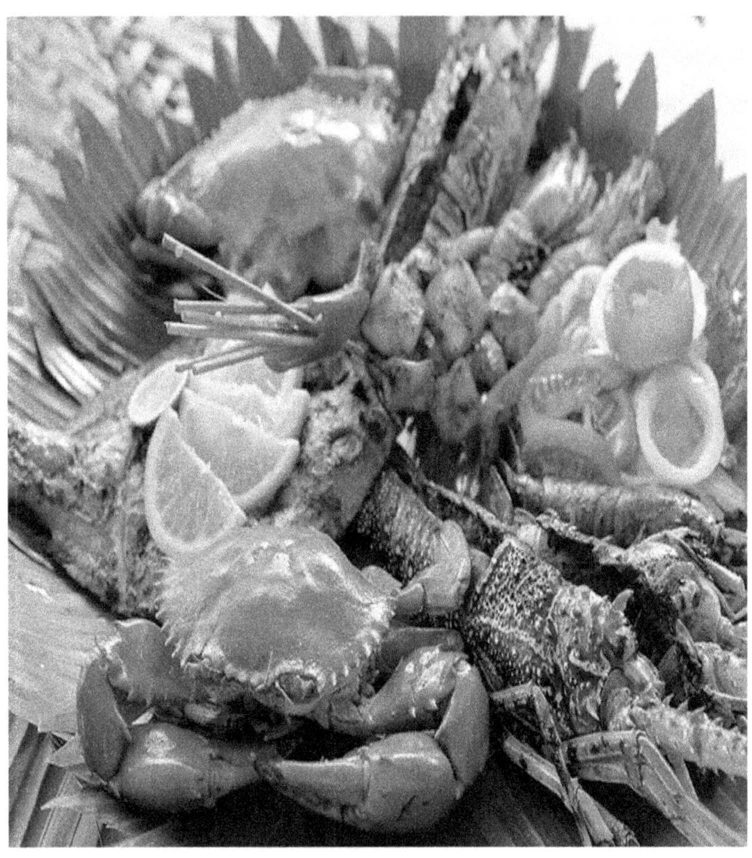

Select a seafood as much as possible

a look and decide which option is best for you before you go. When you arrive at the restaurant, you might ask for no menu, but glancing at the menu at the last minute, will help you resist temptation.

8. Pass on the breadbasket. Please do not place a bread basket on your table. Alternatively, if someone at your table requests it, request a platter of raw vegetables or breadsticks for yourself instead.

9. Avoid the high-end cocktails. If you must have an alcoholic beverage, avoid the cocktail menu; these

beverages are high in sugar and calories, and even one can ruin what could have been a nutritious lunch. Drink a glass of wine, a light beer, a vodka, or a diet tonic instead.

10. Select a seafood dish. Choose a seafood dish, such as white fish, whenever possible. Out of the meat and seafood sections, seafood is the healthiest option.

Just make sure it's not fried and that any condiments are served separately.

11. Drink plenty of water throughout your meal.

This will allow you to savor your food more and ensure that the information that you're full of reaches your brain promptly (before your plate is empty)

12. Skip dessert...do we have to explain why?!!

13. If it's out of sight, it's out of mind

Make the healthy option as simple as possible.

A large component of eating well is having healthful foods readily available.

On the kitchen counter, place a dish of fruit.

Keep any sweets or junk meals in a less visible location.

14. Turn off the television

Television and Internet surfing are both pleasurable and educational pursuits.

However, studies demonstrate that advertisements, product placement, and other promotions that regularly push high-calorie, low-nutrient food and drinks promote unhealthy eating.

Adults should limit their screen usage to no more than 2 hours per day.

Turn off the TV and internet in the children's rooms, and turn them off during mealtime.

15. Snacking at Night

Digestion is a difficult procedure.

Regulate your eating, especially before going to bed, to keep your digestion operating properly.

Your body assumes a calm state during sleep.

It may be impossible to relax if you force it to digest a late dinner.

Experts advise that you avoid eating for at least 2 hours before going to sleep

16. Water Is the Answer!

We should drink 4-6 glasses (2.5 liters) of water each day, according to the guidelines.

Replace your carbonated drinks, juices, and coffee with a glass of plain water.

This will assist to reduce the sugar and calories in these beverages.

Drinking enough water keeps you hydrated, aids digestion, boosts energy levels, and improves the appearance of your skin and hair.

17. distracted Eating

Distractions such as reading the newspaper, watching TV, or texting divert your attention away from eating.

These distractions make determining how full you are more difficult.

You might consume more than you need. Pay attention to what you're eating.

The Cat's Out of the Bag, No.

It's really simple to devour numerous servings without realizing it if you eat straight from the bag.

One of the most important steps in losing weight is to watch what you eat and be conscious of what and how much you're consuming.

Measure out a serving to keep track of your portions.

18. Eating While Running

Eating while driving, at your desk, or on your way out the door.

When you eat on the go, it's all too simple to consume too many calories.

Sitting down to eat can help with this type of eating.

CHAPTER FIVE

The Chinese and Weight Loss

People in China lose weight in a variety of ways.

Eating a lot of acidic, spicy, and bitter meals is good for your health, according to Chinese medicine, because those foods help you lose weight.

Unlike salty, sugary, and fatty foods, which contribute to weight growth Chinese medicine has developed several traditional strategies for losing weight quickly.

Indeed, Chinese medicine advocated a combination of acupuncture, herbs, food restriction, belly massage, and breathing exercises to help patients lose weight by speeding up digestion and treating issues.

Chinese medicine alone is insufficient for weight loss, but when paired with a good diet and physical activity, it can help.

The old-fashioned way

It is quite healthy to consume Chinese plants or drink Chinese herbal tea.

Some Chinese herbs may also aid to curb hunger while also boosting the body's metabolism.

Chi Cao Qian, Fu Ling, and Huang Qi, Bao He Wan are the most well-known brands among Chinese consumers; these Chinese products comprise a range of herbs.

Acupuncture

Acupuncture reduces cravings, boosts energy, improves calm, reduces appetite, and boosts nutrient absorption.

Because the ear contains multiple connecting points that represent most of the major organs and body components, ear acupuncture is regarded as a particularly effective treatment for weight loss.

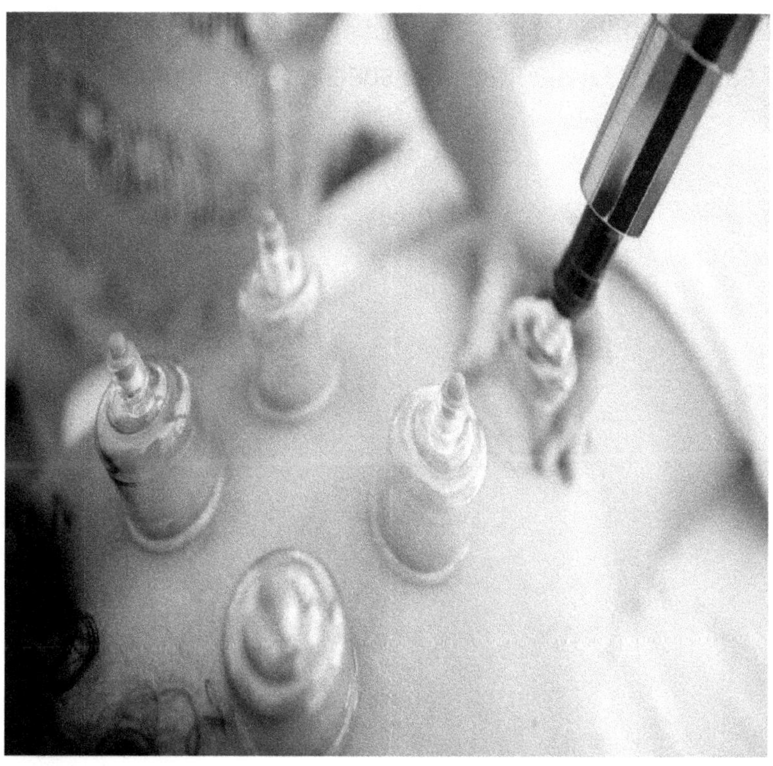

acupuncture reduces cravings, boosts energy, improves calm, reduces appetite, and boosts nutrient absorption.

Acupuncturists occasionally use magnets after each acupuncture treatment or beads on the auricular sites to ensure greater efficiency between sessions.

A comprehensive examination will be required during an acupuncture appointment to determine which points on your body need to be stimulated.

When needles are put into specific important places, the flow of life force known as Qi is improved and restored.

According to Chinese medicine, weight gain can be caused by Qi stagnation in specific regions of the body.

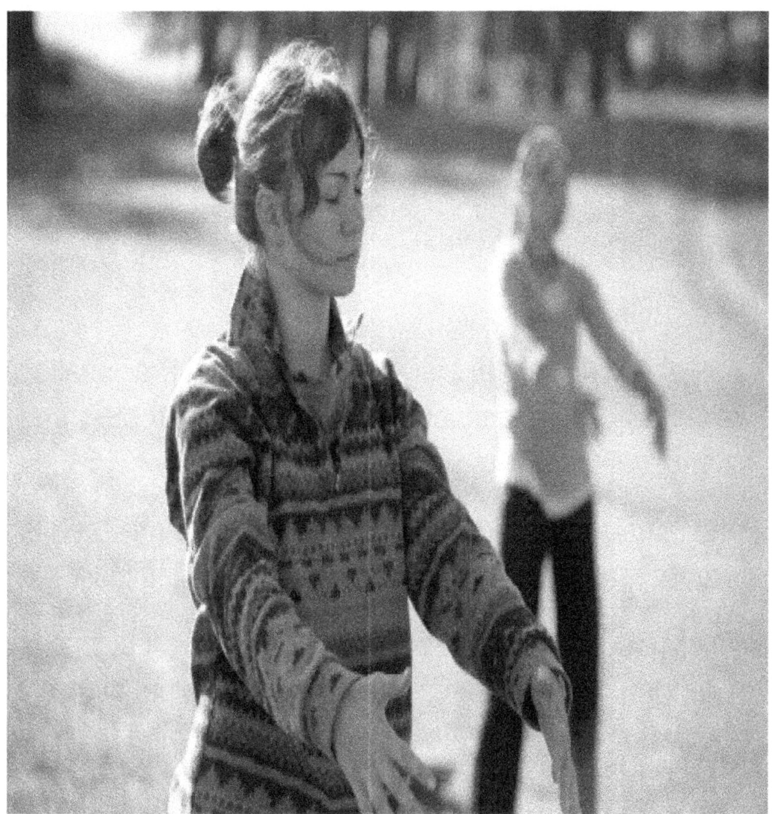

according to Chinese medicine, weight gain can be caused by Qi stagnation in specific regions of the body

Diet Teas

In Chinese culture, tea is very important.

Many studies have demonstrated the health benefits of tea, particularly green tea, a product that is increasingly being offered around the world for its health benefits and weight-loss effects.

Diet teas are made to help you lose weight by removing toxins and waste from your body while also boosting your metabolism.

The way our bodies work is determined by Traditional Chinese Medicine (TCM).

The missing element in the equation is energy.

Indeed, according to Chinese medicine, energy is responsible for our vitality, body control, and overall well-being.

Our ability to shed weight and maintain a healthy weight will be enhanced if this energy is robust and balanced.

Traditional medicine techniques that enhance health include: Meditation is also beneficial for weight loss.

Weight regulation in traditional Chinese medicine is dependent not only on calorie intake and expenditure of energy but also on the focus of Qi maintenance.

The Qi is responsible for increasing your metabolism and making you feel good, according to Chinese medicine.

The Chinese technique of eating foods is well-known for removing toxins and restoring physical equilibrium.

Most detox procedures popular in western cultures, such as drinking green tea or sipping hot lemon water, are well-known in China.

Instead of a rigorous diet, traditional Chinese medicine offers methods for effective detoxification that could provide a quick answer to detoxifying the body and mind.

These approaches are simple to include into our everyday routines to attain long-term improvements, with the primary outcomes being a flatter tummy, improved sleep, better skin, and increased energy levels.

Detoxification with Chinese Tea

Chinese herbs are used to cleanse the kidneys, liver, lungs, and blood.

Regularly drinking tea can help you feel calmer, have more energy, and have cleaner skin.

Many potent herbs are used in the teas, including honeysuckle flower, red clover, dandelion root, and ginger root.

These herbs, when combined, aid in the removal of toxins received by the body from the environment and foods such as pollution, caffeine, smoke, alcohol, and more.

• The Chinese regard Ho Yan Hor Herbal Tea as somewhat of a miracle because of its remarkable ability to heal colds and ease headaches.

Made from a carefully chosen blend of 24 Chinese herbs, each with unique nutritional and therapeutic characteristics.

• Drinking two cups of oolong tea a day can help you burn up to 10% more fat, and it also helps to cleanse your system.

• Green tea is recognized for removing toxins from the body and for containing catechins, an antioxidant that improves liver function.

Cups with suction

Cupping, a painless detoxifying treatment used by the Chinese for hundreds of years, has gained popularity around the world in recent years.

Cupping, like acupuncture, stimulates blood flow and is used to treat infections, colds, and joint and muscle pain.

To generate depression, the practitioner presses glass hard cups straight on your skin. Pumps will allow you to enhance the suction and the amount of skin inside the cup.

Chinese Super Foods

The Chinese use a type of noodle derived from the starch mung bean, which is high in antioxidants.

It is also low in calories and a decent substitute for noodles.

• Pak Choi is a green leaf that promotes digestion and is high in vitamins A and antioxidants. It's one of the most nutrient-dense detox diet meals.

• Sesame seeds have been shown to protect liver cells from the damaging effects of alcohol and other toxins.

Sesame seeds are a great way to cleanse your body.

• Ginger is a potent digestive aid as well as a natural anti-inflammatory and antioxidant powerhouse.

The current weight-loss trend among Chinese consumers

Cleansing juice is one of the Western ways of combating weight gain.

A juice cleanse is a diet consisting entirely of raw fruits and vegetables.

These fluids help the body remove toxins by allowing the digestive system to skip large meals.

pressed increased from zero to around nine businesses on the market throughout those three years.

However, this upward trend has since reversed and many companies have opened physical stores. Proteins are well-known as building blocks for muscles.

Proteins are made up of element combinations of amino acids that join in a variety of ways to form bones, muscles, hair, tendons, skin, and other tissues. They also have other activities, such as enzyme synthesis and nutrient delivery.

Athletes also use protein to repair and rebuild muscle that has been broken down during exercise and to optimize glucose storage as glycogen.

The protein market is expanding as consumers become more concerned about their physical health.

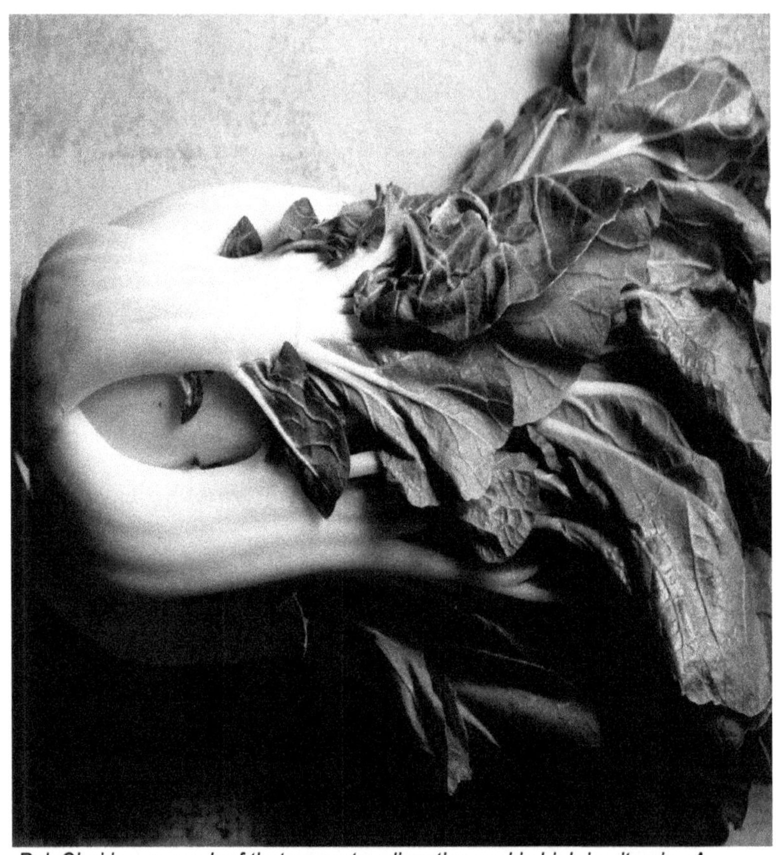

Pak Choi is a green leaf that promotes digestion and is high in vitamins A

Most clients think of the proteins as dietary supplements, and they come in capsule form., pills, powders, granules, and tablets.

Among them are performance enhancers, weight loss, meal replacement powders, and other proteins. Proteins are also used to help people lose weight and to replace meals. These proteins are widely available in China, including fitness clubs and pharmacies., health food stores, and supermarkets, provides consumers with simple access to products and expands the protein market.

There are few native protein powder companies in China, and with the invasion of overseas products, competition is fierce.

Chinese Diet Food Helps You Lose Weight Faster
According to a Chinese proverb, 100% health requires 30% activity and 70% food. It can be observed that a good figure is obtained not only through exercise but also through proper nutrition. Here are some Chinese diet meals that are low in fat, low in calories, and high in fiber, proteins, vitamins, and other nutrients., as well as a one-week Chinese diet plan to help you lose weight quickly and safely.

Cucumber is the number one Chinese diet food.

16 calories/100 grams

Cucumber is high in vitamins and low in calories and contains more than 95% water. The cucumber enzyme found in fresh cucumber can boost human metabolism and blood circulation while also improving the skin's redox effect.

Cucumber with Mashed Garlic, Fried Egg with Cucumbers, and other cucumber-based recipes are recommended.

2. Water Spinach

Calories per 100g: 25

Water spinach has a low-calorie count and can help you lose weight. It's an alkaline vegetable that can help prevent flora imbalance and lessen gut acidity. Niacin and vitamin C are found in water spinach and can help decrease cholesterol and triglycerides. Rich crude cellulose can cause laxation by stimulating intestinal peristalsis and promoting laxation.

Water spinach dishes to try include Water Spinach Boiled, Water Spinach Stir-Fried...

3. Broccoli (30 calories per 100g)

Broccoli has a high fiber content, which allows it to absorb water and swell, making you feel full and allowing you to eat less. Fiber can also aid digestion and absorption, allowing you to eliminate waste more quickly. It's popular Chinese diet food for healthily losing weight.

According to a Japanese study, broccoli has a far higher nutritional content and disease-prevention effect than other vegetables, ranking top. Broccoli has a wide range of nutrients, including protein, carbs, lipids, minerals, vitamin C, and carotene, among others. Broccoli is therefore incredibly healthy.

Broccoli with Garlic, Stir-Fried Broccoli... are some of the recommended broccoli dishes.

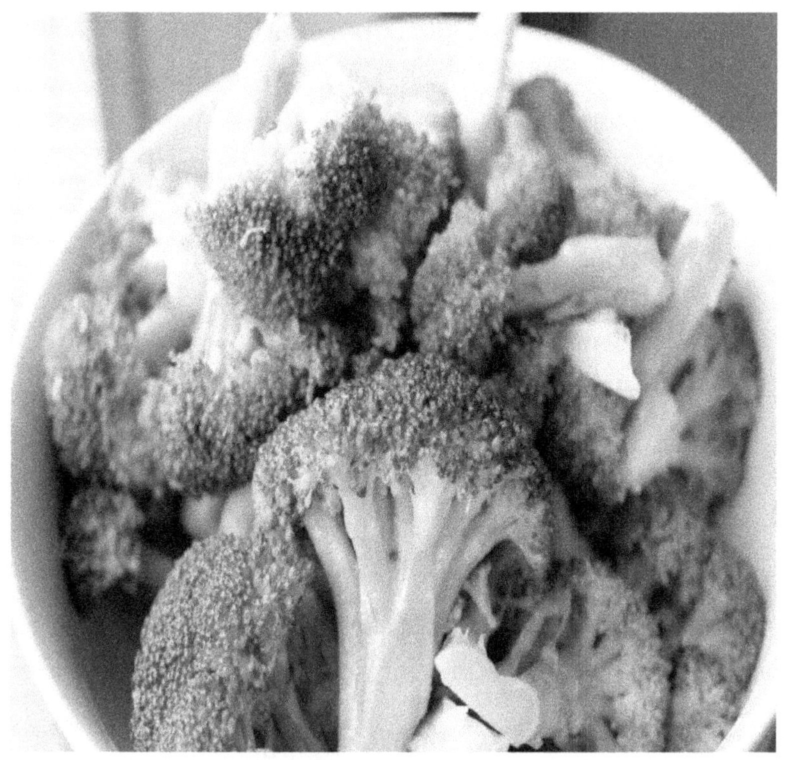

Broccoli is popular Chinese diet food for healthily losing weight

4. Brown Rice (50 calories per 100g)

This is a type of rice that hasn't been processed. It has a higher dietary fiber content than refined rice. Food fiber of this type is insoluble. It will absorb water and expand in the human gut, stimulating stomach motility, reducing constipation, and increasing metabolism. Brown rice is a fantastic everyday dish.

Brown rice meals to try include Steamed Brown Rice, Brown Rice Porridge...

5. Yogurt (60 calories per 100ml) According to one study, persons who consume yogurt lose 61 percent

fatter than those who do not. Yogurt is high in active lactic acid bacteria, which can help to balance flora, enhance gastrointestinal peristalsis, eliminate waste from the gut and relieve constipation. Replacing carbonated drinks with yogurt is sensible for people who are trying to lose weight.

6. Oats (68 calories per 100g)

Oats contain lysine and linoleic acid, which can help lower cholesterol levels in the bloodstream. It also has a high protein content, more than double that of rice, and is the most protein-dense cereal grain. It's not only a great weight-loss diet for teenagers, but it also contains anti-hypertension properties, anti-diabetes, and anti-hyperlipidemia effect in the elderly.

Oatmeal with Milk, Oatmeal Porridge, and other oat-based foods are recommended.

123 calories per 100g of fish

In Chinese cuisine, fish is a delicious and healthy component. Unsaturated fatty acids found in fish can help decrease cholesterol and triglycerides. Fish is high in protein and is easily absorbed by the body. Steaming fish is the greatest technique to cook fish while losing weight because it uses little or no oil.

Steamed Perch, Millet Fish Porridge, and other fish dishes are recommended.

8. Chicken Breast (130 calories per 100g)

Chicken breast is a common ingredient in Chinese cuisine. Among various meats, it is the King of Low-Calorie. Another key quality of Chicken Breast is that it contains no carbohydrates, which is essential for weight loss. The Chicken Breast, on the other hand, is high in protein.

Recommended chicken breast meals include Roasted Chicken Breast, Pan-Fried Chicken Breast...

9. 144 calories for 100g of egg

It's a part of a healthy Chinese diet dish that's high in protein and contains a variety of necessary amino acids. The yolks include lecithin, an emulsifier that breaks down fat and cholesterol into small particles that can be easily removed from the body. Breakfast is best served with an egg.

Egg meals to try to include boiling eggs, steamed eggs, and scrambled eggs with tomatoes...

Green Tea
This tea has 0.5 calories per 100ml of energy.

Green tea contains aromatic components that help to break down fat and prevent it from accumulating in the body. Green tea contains vitamins B1 and C,

	Breakfast	Lunch	Dinner
Monday	One egg, one banana, and 200ml yogurt	One cucumber + 300g pan-fried chicken breast with olive oil	300ml oatmeal+ 300g broccoli + one egg
Tuesday	One corn + 200ml skimmed milk	Two eggs + 300g brown rice porridge with red bean	One apple + 500g steamed fish
Wednesday	300g broccoli + 300 ml millet gruel	200g water spinach + 300g roasted chicken breast + one apple	One egg + one banana + two carrots
Thursday	Six walnuts + one apple + one egg	500g poached fish + 200g water spinach	200ml yogurt with carbohydrates under 10%

Friday	One apple + one banana + one egg	300ml millet gruel + two cucumbers + one egg	Two pieces of oat bread + 200g water spinach + 300g pan-fried chicken breast
Saturday	200ml skimmed milk + one corn + half an apple	300g poached chicken breast + one cucumber + one egg	300ml brown rice porridge with red bean + 200ml low-fat yogurt + two carrots
Sunday	Two steamed eggs + 300g broccoli + one apple	One banana + 500g steamed fish	Two cucumbers + 500g mixed fruit with skimmed milk + two eggs

which encourage the production of gastric juice, and aid digestion and fat elimination. It's an excellent alternative to cola and other high-calorie beverages. Green tea should not be too thick; otherwise, it would obstruct the secretion of gastric juices. On an empty stomach, green tea should not be taken

Chinese Diet for a Week

The key to healthily losing weight is to eat in moderation. Here is a healthy Chinese diet program for you to follow every week meat, grains, vegetables, fruit, dairy products, and other foods that the human body needs.

CHAPTER SIX

Elimination Diet

A food elimination diet is a method of identifying food sensitivities in a methodical manner. There are many different types of food exclusion diets. We eliminated foods that include the eight most frequent allergens from this plan, but you can adjust it as needed if you strongly suspect that, for example, dairy is the problem and prefer to exclusively replace dairy items with non-dairy alternatives.

What is an Elimination Diet?

If you're unsure how to begin an elimination diet, we recommend consulting with a trained dietitian who can assist you through the process safely. They will discuss your current diet and symptoms, as well as assist you in identifying potential food triggers. After that, they will almost certainly advise you to avoid certain trigger foods for at least two weeks, which is where this meal plan might help. This diet can be used as a reference and template for what to eat (or not consume) and can be adjusted to fit your specific needs.

Following the specified elimination period, the reintroduction phase begins, during which you gradually incorporate one suspected food trigger back into your diet. These reintroductions should be spaced out by at least three days to make it easier to figure out which trigger foods produce which symptoms. Keeping a dietary symptom record during this period might be really beneficial. This means you'll keep track of both you are eating habits and your mood.

Dietary Foods to Avoid

The foods to avoid on an elimination diet are highly personalized. The most prevalent food sensitivity is lactose intolerance, some people may wish to start by eliminating lactose, a carbohydrate found in various dairy products. Others believe gluten, a protein found in wheat, is to blame for their problems. The top eight foods most typically associated with food intolerances, sensitivities, and allergies were omitted from this diet.

Milk, as well as dairy products such as yogurt, kefir, butter, cheese, cottage cheese, creamer, half-and-half, sour cream, ice cream, whey or dairy-based powders, as well as any marketed dairy goods, are all examples.

Eggs are used in a variety of meals, including mayonnaise, baked goods, egg-based powders, and more.

Almonds, walnuts, pistachios, cashews, pecans, pralines, pine nuts, and other tree nuts nut milk, nut extracts, and pastes, among other things

Peanut butter, peanut oil, peanut flour, and other products made from peanuts.

Wheat bread, cereal, pasta, breadcrumbs, crackers, flours, and other wheat-based items, as well as bulgur, farro, matzoh meal, seitan, wheatgrass, wheat germ oil, and other wheat-based products.

Soy sauce, tamari, edamame, tofu, tempeh, miso, soymilk, soy yogurt, soy ice cream, soy oil, and other soy products

Salmon, tuna (fresh or tinned), tilapia, bass, anchovies, sardines, haddock, pollock, swordfish, trout, and other types of fish are available.

Crabs, crawfish, lobster, shrimp, prawns, clams, mussels, oysters, scallops, and other shellfish

What Can You Can Eat
While you may have to eliminate a lot of things during an elimination diet, you still get to enjoy a lot of tasty stuff! Here are several examples:

Fruits and vegetables in abundance!

Beans, poultry, and steak are all good sources of protein.

Pumpkin seeds and sunflower butter are good substitutes for nuts.

Quinoa, oats, and corn tortillas are all wheat-free grains.

And plenty of herbs and spices to keep things interesting and tasty.